LOW-IMPACT EXERCISES FOR BALANCE, FLEXIBILITY, AND WELLNESS

CHAIR YOGA FOR SENIORS

JENNIE WAELCHI

Copyright © 2024 by Jennie Waelchi

TABLE OF CONTENTS

INTRODUCTION

Welcome to a transformative journey that will not only change your body but your entire outlook on life. This book is your guide to harnessing the power of chair yoga for weight loss and overall wellness. Whether you are embarking on a weight loss journey for the first time or seeking a new, holistic approach, you are about to embark on a path that nurtures your body, mind, and spirit.

The Power of Chair Yoga

In a world that often moves at breakneck speed, it's easy to overlook the profound benefits of a practice as gentle and accessible as chair yoga. Yet, it's precisely these attributes that make it a powerful tool for weight loss and holistic well-being. Chair yoga is inclusive; it welcomes individuals of all ages, abilities, and fitness levels. The practice recognizes that everybody is unique and that well-being extends beyond the physical.

With chair yoga, you'll discover that weight loss isn't just about shedding pounds; it's about nurturing your body, mind, and soul. It's about developing a harmonious relationship with yourself, understanding your body's cues, and embracing a lifestyle that promotes health and vitality. You're not just on a journey to a slimmer body; you're on a voyage to a more balanced and fulfilling life.

The Structure of This Book

This book is structured to guide you through a comprehensive chair yoga program for weight loss and wellness. Each chapter builds upon the previous one, creating a strong foundation for your journey.

Your Transformation Awaits

Through each chapter, you'll not only build physical strength and flexibility but also cultivate mindfulness and self-awareness. You'll develop a profound mind-body connection that extends far beyond the confines of your yoga mat.

As you embrace the practice of chair yoga, you'll realize that weight loss is not a destination; it's a journey of self-discovery, resilience, and growth. Your body is your faithful companion on this journey, and chair yoga is the key that unlocks its potential.

So, welcome to a world of weight loss wisdom through chair yoga. The experience starts, and the potential outcomes are huge. The power to transform your life is in your hands, and the wisdom to do so is within these pages. We ought to set out on this historic trip together.

Welcome to the World of Chair Yoga

In the hustle and bustle of our modern lives, where time seems to slip through our fingers and the demands on our bodies and minds are ever-increasing, we often forget to take a moment for ourselves. We forget to breathe, to stretch, and to nurture our inner selves. In this fast-paced world, finding time for physical fitness and mental well-being can feel like an insurmountable challenge. This is where chair yoga comes to the rescue, offering you a tranquil sanctuary within the chaos of everyday life.

A Path to Wellness and Transformation

Chair yoga is not merely a practice; it's a holistic approach to wellness and transformation. It invites you to embark on a journey that nourishes your body, calms your mind, and awakens your spirit. It extends an invitation to individuals of all ages and abilities to experience the profound benefits of yoga in a way that is gentle, accessible, and profoundly empowering.

As you enter the world of chair yoga, you step onto a path that leads to greater physical health, mental clarity, and emotional balance. This path is designed to be inclusive, ensuring that regardless of your age, fitness level, or physical abilities, you can partake in the boundless advantages of yoga. It recognizes the uniqueness of your body, acknowledging that every person is an individual with distinct needs and goals. Chair yoga offers you the wisdom and tools to nurture your body and embark on a voyage of transformation.

Chair Yoga: A Practice for Everyone

One of the remarkable attributes of chair yoga is its universal appeal. Whether you're a seasoned yogi or brand new to the practice, whether you're in the prime of life or your golden years, chair yoga welcomes you with open arms. It's a practice that knows no boundaries and recognizes no limitations.

For those who have struggled to find a fitness routine that suits their physical condition or lifestyle, chair yoga offers a versatile solution. It can be practiced in the comfort of your home or office, with nothing more than a sturdy chair as your faithful companion. It is an antidote to the sedentary nature of modern life, a bridge to greater mobility and strength.

The Journey Begins

As you turn the pages of this book and explore the world of chair yoga, you will unlock the secrets to a healthier, more balanced life. You will learn how to harness the power of your breath, how to savor each bite with mindful eating, and how to enhance your flexibility and strength. Chair yoga will guide you toward a deeper connection with your body and foster mindfulness, empowering you to make healthier choices and embrace a lifestyle that promotes vitality and well-being.

This journey is not just about losing weight; it's about finding yourself. It's about cultivating a relationship with your body that is built on love, compassion, and self-acceptance. It's about recognizing that wellness is not a destination but an ongoing path of growth and self-discovery.

As you embark on this adventure, remember that the power to transform your life resides within you. Chair yoga is merely the compass, pointing you in the direction of a more balanced, fulfilled existence. The possibilities are infinite, and the journey is bound to be extraordinary. So, welcome to the world of chair yoga, where the adventure begins, and the transformation awaits.

Understanding the Connection Between Yoga and Weight Loss

The relationship between yoga and weight loss may not be immediately apparent, as yoga is often associated with relaxation, mindfulness, and flexibility rather than intense physical exercise. However, the practice of yoga can play a significant role in a weight loss journey when approached mindfully and holistically. In this exploration, we will delve into the various ways in which yoga and weight loss are interconnected, emphasizing the importance of the mind-body connection in achieving sustainable results.

Mindful Eating and Weight Management

One of the most direct connections between yoga and weight loss is through mindful eating. Yoga promotes a heightened awareness of the body's sensations, including hunger and fullness cues. This awareness is central to mindful eating, a practice that encourages you to savor every bite, eat with intention, and listen to your body's needs.

By practicing mindful eating, you become attuned to when you're truly hungry and when you're satisfied. This can forestall indulging, profound eating, and careless nibbling, which are normal supporters of weight gain. The mindfulness cultivated through yoga extends into your eating habits, helping you make better food choices and fostering a healthier relationship with food.

Stress Reduction and Emotional Eating

Stress is a significant factor in weight gain and difficulty in losing weight. High-feelings of anxiety can set off close to home eating, where people go to nourishment for solace or interruption. Yoga is renowned for its stress-reduction benefits, as it encourages relaxation, deep breathing, and the release of tension.

Yoga practices, particularly those that involve deep breathing and meditation, activate the body's relaxation response. This reduces the production of stress hormones, such as cortisol, which can lead to cravings for unhealthy, high-calorie foods. By managing stress through yoga, you are less likely to turn to emotional eating as a coping mechanism, thereby supporting your weight loss goals.

Physical Activity and Caloric Expenditure

While yoga is often associated with gentle movements and stretching, it can be a valuable component of a weight loss strategy. Many forms of yoga, such as Vinyasa or Power Yoga, are physically demanding and can provide a cardiovascular workout that burns calories.

Moreover, building lean muscle through yoga can boost your metabolism. Muscle tissue burns more calories at rest than fat tissue, so the more muscle you have, the more calories you burn, even when you're not actively exercising. Additionally, regular yoga practice can increase your overall physical activity level and energy expenditure, contributing to weight loss.

Enhanced Metabolism and Digestion

Certain yoga poses and sequences stimulate the endocrine system, particularly the thyroid gland, which plays a crucial role in metabolism regulation. A balanced thyroid function supports the efficient conversion of food into energy, which can aid in weight management.

Yoga also promotes healthy digestion by massaging and stimulating the digestive organs. Poses that involve twists and stretches can alleviate bloating and discomfort, ensuring that the body absorbs nutrients effectively. A healthy digestive system can lead to better nutrient absorption and the prevention of weight gain due to nutrient deficiencies.

Building Body Awareness and Self-Compassion

Perhaps one of the most profound connections between yoga and weight loss lies in the development of body awareness and self-compassion. Yoga encourages you to listen to your body's signals, embrace its limitations, and cultivate a loving and respectful relationship with it. This mindset shift is instrumental in a successful weight loss journey.

When you are in tune with your body's needs, you are more likely to make choices that support your well-being. You'll know when you need nourishing food, exercise, rest, or self-care. You'll also develop self-compassion, which allows you to approach your weight loss journey with kindness rather than self-criticism. This shift in perspective can be transformative, as it reduces the stress and emotional burden often associated with weight loss efforts.

Holistic Well-Being and Weight Loss

Yoga, at its core, is a practice that fosters holistic well-being. It goes beyond the physical aspects and touches upon mental, emotional, and spiritual dimensions. By addressing the entirety of your well-being, yoga supports a comprehensive approach to weight loss. It encourages you to not only shed pounds but also to gain vitality, balance, and self-awareness.

The connection between yoga and weight loss is multifaceted. The practice of yoga enhances mindful eating, reduces stress, and supports emotional well-being. It also contributes to physical activity and calorie expenditure, while improving metabolism and digestion. However, the most profound impact is in the development of body awareness and self-compassion, which creates a solid foundation for sustainable weight loss and a lifelong journey to well-being. Yoga is not just a weight loss tool; it's a pathway to a healthier, more fulfilling life.

CHAPTER ONE

THE FOUNDATIONS OF CHAIR YOGA

Exploring the Basics of Chair Yoga

Chair yoga is a gentle, accessible form of yoga that can be practiced by individuals of all ages and physical abilities. In this chapter, we'll explore the fundamental principles and techniques that form the basis of chair yoga. By understanding these foundational elements, you'll be better equipped to embark on your journey towards weight loss and improved well-being through chair yoga.

The Essence of Chair Yoga

Chair yoga, as the name suggests, is a variation of traditional yoga that incorporates a chair into the practice. Unlike traditional yoga, which often involves complex poses and stretches on a yoga mat, chair yoga is performed while seated on a chair or using a chair for support. The chair becomes a stable and secure prop, making yoga accessible to a wide range of individuals, including those with limited mobility, injuries, or health conditions.

One of the key features of chair yoga is that it is adaptable to the needs of the individual. Whether you're a complete beginner or an experienced yogi, chair yoga can be tailored to your specific level of comfort and fitness. It's an excellent option for seniors, people recovering from injuries, or anyone looking for a gentle way to stay active and promote physical and mental well-being.

The Benefits of Chair Yoga for Weight Loss

You might be wondering how a practice that involves sitting on a chair can contribute to weight loss. While chair yoga may not be as intense as some other forms of exercise, it offers a holistic approach to well-being that can support your weight loss goals in several ways.

1. **Enhanced Awareness**: Chair yoga places a strong emphasis on mindfulness and body awareness. As you practice, you become more attuned to your body's sensations, your posture, and your breath. This heightened awareness can extend to your eating habits, helping you recognize hunger and fullness cues and make better choices about what and when to eat.

2. **Stress Reduction**: Stress is a common contributor to weight gain. Chair yoga incorporates relaxation and stress-reduction techniques, which can help manage stress and reduce emotional eating. You'll learn to use your breath to calm your mind and body, making it easier to make mindful choices when it comes to food.

3. **Improved Metabolism**: While chair yoga may not be an intense calorie-burning exercise, it can help improve circulation and stimulate your metabolism. Regular practice can assist in maintaining a healthy metabolic rate, which is essential for sustainable weight loss.

4. **Strength and Flexibility**: Chair yoga includes gentle movements and stretches that promote strength and flexibility. As your muscle tone increases and your joints become more supple, you'll find it easier to engage in other physical activities that support weight loss, such as walking or more vigorous forms of exercise.

5. **Posture and Core Strengthening**: Good posture is essential for overall well-being, and it can also make you appear taller and leaner. Chair yoga exercises can help you maintain a strong core and improve your posture, which can have a positive impact on your self-esteem and the way you carry yourself.

Choosing the Right Chair and Setting Up Your Space

Before you dive into chair yoga practice, it's essential to select the right chair and create a suitable space for your sessions.

Selecting the Right Chair

The ideal chair for chair yoga is stable, sturdy, and comfortable. Here are some tips to consider when choosing a chair:

1. **Stability**: Ensure that the chair is solid and does not wobble. It should be able to support your weight without any concerns.

2. **Backrest**: A chair with a straight backrest is preferable for most chair yoga poses. However, if you

have specific back issues, a chair with a slightly reclined backrest may be more comfortable.

3. **Armrests**: While armrests can be helpful for balance and support, some poses may require you to have access to the sides of the chair without obstruction. A chair with removable or adjustable armrests can be an excellent choice.

4. **Seat Height**: The height of the chair should allow your feet to rest flat on the floor with your knees at a 90-degree angle. If your chair is too high, you can use a cushion or yoga block to raise the floor level.

5. **Comfort**: Look for a chair with a cushioned seat that provides comfort during prolonged sessions. You may also want to use a cushion or blanket on the chair for added comfort, especially if you have sensitive joints.

Once you've chosen the right chair, you're ready to set up your chair yoga space.

Creating a Comfortable Space

Having a dedicated and inviting space for your chair yoga practice can enhance your overall experience. This is the way you can make an optimal space:

1. **Clear the Area**: Ensure that the space around your chair is clear of any obstacles or tripping hazards. You should be able to move your arms and legs freely during the practice.

2. **Lighting**: Use natural or soft artificial lighting to create a soothing atmosphere. Harsh lighting can be distracting, so opt for a warm and inviting ambiance.

3. **Comfortable Clothing**: Wear comfortable, loose-fitting clothing that allows you to move freely. You don't need any specialized yoga attire for chair yoga — the key is to feel at ease in what you're wearing.

4. **Breathable Flooring**: If you're practicing chair yoga on a hard surface, consider using a yoga mat or a non-slip rug underneath your chair to enhance comfort and stability.

5. **Accessories**: Gather any props or accessories you may need for your practice, such as a cushion, blanket, or yoga block. These can be used to modify poses and enhance your comfort.

As you prepare your chair and space, remember that chair yoga is all about adaptability. It's perfectly fine to experiment with different setups until you find what works best for you. The most important thing is that you feel secure, comfortable, and ready to embark on your chair yoga journey.

CHAPTER TWO

BASIC CHAIR YOGA POSES

In this chapter, you'll learn a variety of basic chair yoga poses designed to improve flexibility, strength, and balance while providing a gentle and accessible practice for seniors. These poses form the foundation of your chair yoga journey and can be modified to suit your needs. We will cover warm-up poses, seated breathing exercises, arm and shoulder stretches, leg and hip stretches, and neck and spine stretches.

Warm-Up Poses

Before diving into specific poses, it's important to begin your practice with gentle warm-up exercises. These movements help prepare your body for the practice and prevent injury.

1. **Seated Cat-Cow Stretch:**

    - Begin seated with your back straight and your feet flat on the floor, hip-width apart.

    - Place your hands on your thighs.

    - Inhale and arch your back, lifting your chest and tilting your head back slightly (Cow Pose).

    - • Breathe out and adjust your spine, tucking your jaw to your chest (Feline Posture).

    - Repeat for several breaths, moving slowly and gently.

2. **Seated Side Bends:**

- Sit upright in your chair with your feet on the floor and hands resting on your thighs.

- • Breathe in and raise your left arm above, coming to towards the right side.

- Exhale and gently bend your torso to the right, keeping your left sit bone grounded.

- Hold for a couple of breaths, then, at that point, return to the middle.

- Repeat on the other side, raising your right arm overhead and bending to the left.

- Perform 3-5 sets on each side.

3. **Seated Torso Twists:**

- Sit upright with your feet flat on the floor and hands resting on your thighs.

- Place your right hand on the back of the chair and your left hand on the outside of your right thigh.

- Inhale and lengthen your spine.

- Exhale and gently twist your torso to the right, keeping your back straight.

- Hold for a couple of breaths, then, at that point, return to the middle.

- Rehash on the opposite side, turning to one side.

- Perform 3-5 sets on each side.

Seated Breathing Exercises

Breathing exercises are an essential part of yoga practice, helping to calm the mind and improve focus. Here are two breathing exercises you can practice while seated:

1. **Diaphragmatic Breathing:**

   - Sit comfortably in your chair with your back straight and feet on the floor.

   - Put one hand on your chest and the other on your mid-region.

   - Breathe in leisurely through your nose, permitting your mid-region to ascend as you fill your lungs with air.

   - Breathe out leisurely through your mouth, feeling your mid-region fall.

   - Focus on keeping your chest relatively still and breathing from your diaphragm.

   - Repeat for several breaths, aiming for slow, steady inhales and exhales.

2. **Alternate Nostril Breathing:**

- Sit upright in your chair and rest your left hand on your left thigh.

- Use your right thumb to close your right nostril.

- Inhale through your left nostril.

- • Close your left nostril with your right ring finger and delivery your thumb from your right nostril.

- Exhale through your right nostril.

- Inhale through your right nostril.

- Close your right nostril with your right thumb and release your ring finger from your left nostril.

- Exhale through your left nostril.

- Repeat this cycle for several breaths.

Arm and Shoulder Stretches

Arm and shoulder stretches help release tension in the upper body and improve flexibility.

1. **Seated Arm Circles:**

- • Sit with your back straight and feet on the floor.

- Extend your arms out to the sides, parallel to the floor.

- Slowly make small circles with your arms, starting with forward circles.

- Continue for 10-15 seconds, then reverse direction and circle backward.

- Perform 2-3 sets in each direction.

2. **Eagle Arms:**

   - Sit upright in your chair.

   - Cross your right arm over your left, bending your elbows and bringing your forearms together.

   - Try to touch your palms or the backs of your hands together.

   - Lift your elbows slightly and hold the stretch for a few breaths.

   - Release and repeat on the other side, crossing your left arm over your right.

   - Perform 2-3 sets on each side.

3. **Seated Shoulder Rolls:**

   - Sit upright in your chair with your back straight.

- Inhale and roll your shoulders up towards your ears.

- Exhale and roll your shoulders back and down.

- Repeat the movement for several breaths, and then reverse direction (forward rolls).

- Perform 2-3 sets in each direction.

Leg and Hip Stretches

Leg and hip stretches improve flexibility and range of motion in the lower body.

1. **Seated Knee-to-Chest Stretch:**

   - Sit in your chair with your back straight and feet on the floor.

   - Lift your right leg and hug your knee to your chest.

   - Hold the stretch for a few breaths, then release and lower your foot back to the floor.

   - Repeat with your left leg.

   - Perform 3-5 sets on each side.

2. **Seated Figure Four Stretch:**

   - Sit with your back straight and feet on the floor.

- Cross your right ankle over your left knee, creating a "figure four" shape with your legs.

- Tenderly press your right knee down to extend the stretch.

- Hold for a couple of breaths, then, at that point, delivery and switch sides.

- Perform 3-5 sets on each side.

3. **Seated Calf Stretch:**

- Sit with your back straight and feet on the floor.

- Extend your right leg straight and flex your foot towards your shin.

- Hold for a few breaths, then point your foot away from your body and hold.

- Repeat with your left leg.

- Perform 3-5 sets on each side.

Neck and Spine Stretches

Neck and spine extends assist with alleviating strain and further develop portability in the chest area.

1. **Seated Neck Stretch:**

- Sit upstanding in your seat.

- Gradually slant your head to one side, bringing your right ear towards your right shoulder.
- Hold for a couple of breaths, then, at that point, return to the middle and slant your head to one side.
- Perform 3-5 sets on each side.

2.   Seated Spinal Turn:

- Sit in your seat with your back straight and feet on the floor.
- Put your left hand outwardly of your right thigh and your right hand on the rear of your seat.
- Breathe in and protract your spine, then breathe out and delicately wind to one side.
- Hold for a couple of breaths, then return to the middle and switch sides.
- Perform 3-5 sets on each side.

3.   Seated Forward Crease:

- Sit with your back straight and feet on the floor.
- Breathe in and extend your spine.
- Breathe out and pivot forward from your hips, coming to towards your feet or the floor.
- Hold for a couple of breaths, then leisurely roll back up to a situated position.
- Perform 3-5 sets.

These fundamental seat yoga presents offer a delicate yet viable prologue to your training. By integrating these activities into your daily schedule, you can further develop adaptability, strength, and equilibrium while encountering the quieting impacts of yoga. Make sure to pay attention to your body and alter acts like required. Practice consistently and partake in the advantages of seat yoga as you progress. In the following section, you'll investigate seat yoga streams that consolidate these postures into groupings for a balanced practice. We should proceed with your excursion to health!

CHAPTER THREE

CHAIR YOGA FLOWS

Chair yoga flows are sequences of poses linked together to create a seamless and fluid practice. These flows can be tailored to your individual needs and goals, whether you're seeking energy and vitality, relaxation and stress relief, balance and stability, or flexibility and mobility. In this chapter, we'll explore a variety of chair yoga flows that incorporate the basic poses you've learned in the previous chapter. These flows are designed to enhance your practice and improve your overall well-being.

Flow for Energy and Vitality

This flow focuses on invigorating the body and mind by increasing blood circulation and energizing the muscles. It's an extraordinary method for beginning your day or lift your energy levels.

1. **Seated Cat-Cow Stretch:**

   - Begin with seated cat-cow stretches to warm up your spine. Inhale as you arch your back and lift your chest (Cow Pose), then exhale as you round your spine and tuck your chin (Cat Pose).

   - Repeat for 5 breaths.

2. **Seated Arm Circles:**

- Move into arm circles by extending your arms out to the sides and making forward circles with your arms for 10-15 seconds.

- Reverse direction and circle backward for 10-15 seconds.

3. **Seated Side Bends:**

- Sit upright and reach your left arm overhead.

- Gently bend to the right, holding the stretch for a few breaths.

- Repeat on the other side.

- Perform 3 sets on each side.

4. **Seated Knee-to-Chest Stretch:**

- Lift your right leg and hug your knee to your chest, holding for a few breaths.

- Repeat with your left leg.

- Perform 3 sets on each side.

5. **Seated Figure Four Stretch:**

- Cross your right ankle over your left knee.

- Hold the stretch for a few breaths.

- Repeat on the other side.

- Perform 3 sets on each side.

6. **Seated Forward Fold:**

   - Pivot forward from your hips, coming to towards your feet or the floor.

   - Hold the posture for a couple of breaths.

   - Slowly roll back up to a seated position.

7. **Seated Breathing Exercise:**

   - Finish the flow with diaphragmatic breathing for 1-2 minutes.

Flow for Relaxation and Stress Relief

This flow focuses on calming the mind and body through gentle movements and deep breathing exercises. It's perfect for unwinding at the end of the day or whenever you need to relax.

1. **Seated Neck Stretch:**

   - Start with seated neck stretches, tilting your head to each side for 3-5 breaths.

   - Perform 3 sets on each side.

2. **Seated Shoulder Rolls:**

   - • Roll your shoulders up towards your ears and afterward back and down.

- Repeat for 5 breaths in each direction.

3. **Seated Torso Twists:**

   - • Bend your middle to one side, holding for a couple of breaths.

   - Repeat on the other side.

   - Perform 3 sets on each side.

4. **Seated Figure Four Stretch:**

   - Cross your right ankle over your left knee and hold the stretch for a few breaths.

   - Repeat on the other side.

   - Perform 3 sets on each side.

5. **Seated Cat-Cow Stretch:**

   - Move into seated cat-cow stretches, alternating between arching and rounding your spine.

   - Repeat for 5 breaths.

6. **Seated Forward Fold:**

   - Hinge forward from your hips and reach towards your feet or the floor.

   - Hold the pose for several breaths.

   - Slowly roll back up to a seated position.

7. **Alternate Nostril Breathing:**

- Finish the flow with alternate nostril breathing for 1-2 minutes.

Flow for Balance and Stability

This flow targets balance and stability through exercises that engage your core and strengthen your legs. Practicing this flow regularly can help prevent falls and improve your overall mobility.

1. **Seated Knee-to-Chest Stretch:**

- Lift your right leg and hug your knee to your chest, holding for a few breaths.

- Repeat with your left leg.

- Perform 3 sets on each side.

2. **Seated Leg Extensions:**

- Extend your right leg straight and hold for a few breaths.

- Repeat with your left leg.

- Perform 3 sets on each side.

3. **Seated Heel-to-Toe Walk:**

- • Place your right foot before your left, impact point to toe.

- Hold the position for a few breaths, then switch legs.

- Perform 3 sets on each side.

4. **Seated Ankle Circles:**

   - Lift your right leg slightly and circle your ankle in one direction for 10-15 seconds.

   - Reverse direction and repeat.

   - Perform 2-3 sets on each side.

5. **Seated Hip Circles:**

   - Lift your right knee and circle your leg in one direction for 10-15 seconds.

   - Reverse direction and repeat.

   - Perform 2-3 sets on each side.

6. **Seated Torso Twists:**

   - Curve your middle to one side, holding for a couple of breaths.

   - Repeat on the other side.

   - Perform 3 sets on each side.

7. **Seated Breathing Exercise:**

   - Finish the flow with diaphragmatic breathing for 1-2 minutes.

Flow for Flexibility and Mobility

This flow focuses on improving flexibility and mobility through gentle stretches for your entire body.

1. **Seated Side Bends:**

   - Begin with seated side bends, reaching your arm overhead and bending to each side.

   - Hold each stretch for 3-5 breaths.

   - Perform 3 sets on each side.

2. **Seated Forward Fold:**

   - Hinge forward from your hips and reach towards your feet or the floor.

   - Hold the pose for several breaths.

   - Slowly roll back up to a seated position.

3. **Seated Cat-Cow Stretch:**

   - Move into seated cat-cow stretches, alternating between arching and rounding your spine.

   - Repeat for 5 breaths.

4. **Seated Knee-to-Chest Stretch:**

   - Lift your right leg and hug your knee to your chest, holding for a few breaths.

   - Repeat with your left leg.

- Perform 3 sets on each side.

5. **Seated Figure Four Stretch:**

   - Cross your right ankle over your left knee and hold the stretch for a few breaths.

   - Repeat on the other side.

   - Perform 3 sets on each side.

6. **Seated Spinal Twist:**

   - Curve your middle to one side, holding for a couple of breaths.

   - Repeat on the other side.

   - Perform 3 sets on each side.

7. **Alternate Nostril Breathing:**

   - Finish the flow with alternate nostril breathing for 1-2 minutes.

Chair yoga flows allow you to practice a variety of poses in a smooth and fluid sequence, targeting different areas of the body and promoting overall well-being. Whether you're looking for energy, relaxation, balance, or flexibility, these flows provide a comprehensive practice that can be tailored to your individual needs. Remember to listen to your body and modify the flows as needed. In the next chapter, you'll explore how chair yoga can be used to address common ailments and improve your quality of life. Let's continue your journey to wellness!

CHAPTER FOUR

CHAIR YOGA FOR COMMON AILMENTS

Chair yoga can be a powerful tool for managing and improving a variety of common ailments that affect seniors. Through gentle movements and mindful breathing, chair yoga can alleviate symptoms, improve function, and enhance quality of life. In this chapter, we'll explore how chair yoga can address specific conditions such as arthritis, back pain, circulatory issues, digestive health, and respiratory health. For each ailment, we'll provide an overview, followed by chair yoga practices that may help improve the condition.

Yoga for Arthritis Relief

Joint pain is a typical condition that influences the joints, causing torment, solidness, and decreased versatility. Chair yoga can help manage arthritis by gently moving the joints, increasing flexibility, and reducing inflammation.

1. **Seated Finger and Wrist Stretches:**

   - Begin seated with your back straight and feet flat on the floor.

   - Extend your arms forward and spread your fingers apart.

   - Close your fists and then open your hands wide, repeating the movement several times.

- Perform wrist circles by rotating your wrists in both directions for 10-15 seconds each.

- Repeat 2-3 times.

2. **Seated Shoulder Rolls:**

   - • Roll your shoulders up towards your ears and afterward back and down.

   - Perform forward and backward rolls for 10-15 seconds in each direction.

   - Repeat 2-3 times.

3. **Seated Ankle Circles:**

   - Lift your right foot off the floor and circle your ankle in one direction for 10-15 seconds.

   - Reverse direction and repeat.

   - Repeat with your left ankle.

   - Perform 2-3 sets on each side.

4. **Seated Knee-to-Chest Stretch:**

   - Lift your right knee to your chest and hug it gently, holding the stretch for a few breaths.

   - Repeat with your left knee.

   - Perform 3-5 sets on each side.

5. **Seated Forward Fold:**

- Hinge forward from your hips and reach towards your feet.

- Hold the stretch for several breaths.

- Slowly roll back up to a seated position.

6. **Seated Spinal Twist:**

- • Curve your middle to one side, holding for a couple of breaths.

- Repeat on the other side.

- Perform 3 sets on each side.

Yoga for Back Pain Management

Back pain is a common complaint, often caused by poor posture, muscle strain, or underlying conditions such as herniated discs. Chair yoga can provide relief by stretching and strengthening the muscles that support the spine.

1. **Seated Cat-Cow Stretch:**

- Begin with seated cat-cow stretches to gently move your spine.

- Inhale as you arch your back (Cow Pose), then exhale as you round your spine (Cat Pose).

- Repeat for 5 breaths.

2. **Seated Side Bends:**

   - Reach your left arm overhead and bend to the right, holding the stretch for a few breaths.

   - Repeat on the other side.

   - Perform 3 sets on each side.

3. **Seated Torso Twists:**

   - • Curve your middle to one side and hold for a couple of breaths.

   - Repeat on the other side.

   - Perform 3 sets on each side.

4. **Seated Forward Fold:**

   - Hinge forward from your hips and reach towards your feet or the floor.

   - Hold for several breaths.

   - Slowly roll back up to a seated position.

5. **Seated Hip Stretch:**

   - Cross your right ankle over your left knee and hold the stretch for a few breaths.

   - Repeat on the other side.

   - Perform 3 sets on each side.

Yoga for Improved Circulation

Good circulation is essential for overall health, as it delivers oxygen and nutrients to the body's cells. Chair yoga can enhance circulation by gently moving the body and encouraging blood flow.

1. **Seated Ankle Circles:**

   - Lift your right foot off the floor and circle your ankle in one direction for 10-15 seconds.

   - Reverse direction and repeat.

   - Repeat with your left ankle.

   - Perform 2-3 sets on each side.

2. **Seated Leg Extensions:**

   - Extend your right leg straight and hold for a few breaths.

   - Repeat with your left leg.

   - Perform 3 sets on each side.

3. **Seated Heel-to-Toe Walk:**

   - Place your right foot before your left, impact point to toe.

   - Walk your feet forward in this manner for several steps, then walk backward.

- Perform 3-5 sets.

4. **Seated Arm Circles:**

   - Extend your arms out to the sides and make small circles for 10-15 seconds.

   - Reverse direction and repeat.

   - Perform 2-3 sets in each direction.

5. **Seated Breathing Exercises:**

   - Practice diaphragmatic breathing or alternate nostril breathing for 1-2 minutes.

Yoga for Digestive Health

Chair yoga can improve digestion by stimulating the digestive system and encouraging the movement of food through the body.

1. **Seated Torso Twists:**

   - Begin with seated torso twists, gently twisting to each side.

   - Hold the stretch for a few breaths on each side.

   - Perform 3 sets on each side.

2. **Seated Side Bends:**

   - Reach your arm overhead and bend to the opposite side, holding the stretch for a few breaths.

   - Repeat on the other side.

   - Perform 3 sets on each side.

3. **Seated Knee-to-Chest Stretch:**

   - Lift your right knee to your chest and hug it gently.

   - Repeat with your left knee.

   - Perform 3-5 sets on each side.

4. **Seated Forward Fold:**

   - Hinge forward from your hips and reach towards your feet or the floor.

   - Hold the stretch for several breaths.

   - Slowly roll back up to a seated position.

5. **Seated Cat-Cow Stretch:**

   - Alternate between arching and rounding your spine, moving slowly and mindfully.

   - Repeat for 5 breaths.

Yoga for Respiratory Wellbeing

Seat yoga can upgrade respiratory wellbeing by further developing lung limit and empowering profound, careful relaxing.

1.   Seated Breathing Activities:

- Practice diaphragmatic relaxing for 1-2 minutes.
- You can likewise attempt substitute nostril relaxing for another 1-2 minutes.

2.   Seated Side Twists:

- Arrive at your arm above and twist aside.

- Hold for a couple of breaths on each side.

- Perform 3 sets on each side.

3.   Seated Arm Circles:

- Stretch out your arms out to the sides and circle them toward every path for 10-15 seconds.
- Perform 2-3 sets toward every path.

4.   Seated Chest Opener:

- Place your hands behind your back and catch them together.
- Lift your chest and tenderly curve your back.
- Hold the stretch for a couple of breaths, then, at that point, discharge.

5.   **Seated Spinal Contort:**

•   Contort your middle to each side, holding the stretch for a couple of breaths.

•   Perform 3 sets on each side.

Seat yoga offers a protected and compelling method for overseeing and further develop normal diseases like joint inflammation, back torment, circulatory issues, stomach related wellbeing, and respiratory wellbeing. By integrating designated seat yoga practices into your daily schedule, you can encounter alleviation from side effects and improve your general personal satisfaction. Make sure to pay attention to your body and change acts like required. In the following section, we'll investigate further developed seat yoga practices and how to coordinate props and adornments into your daily schedule for added help. We should proceed with your excursion to health!

High level Seat YOGA PRACTICES AND THE Utilization OF PROPS

In this part, you will investigate further developed seat yoga practices and how to consolidate different props and accomplices to upgrade your training. By figuring out how to coordinate props, for example, yoga lashes, blocks, and opposition groups, you can develop your stretches, work on your arrangement, and designer your training to your singular requirements.

Outline:

•	High level Seat Yoga Practices: This segment presents really testing seat yoga postures and successions to upgrade strength, adaptability, and equilibrium.

•	Props and Frill: Figure out how to utilize props, for example, yoga lashes, blocks, and opposition groups to alter stances and backing your training.

•	Seat Yoga Streams with Props: Consolidate progressed postures and props in streaming successions for a complete practice.

•	Redoing Seat Yoga: Find ways of altering your seat yoga practice in light of your particular objectives, requirements, and impediments.

High level Seat Yoga Practices

Integrate progressed stances and successions into your seat yoga practice to extend your training and challenge your body.

### 1.	Seated Champion II:

- Sit sideways on your seat, left leg bowed at a 90-degree point, right leg stretched out straight out aside.
- Raise your arms to bear level, one arm arriving at forward and the other back, palms dealing with.

- Hold the posture for a few breaths, then switch sides.

2. **Seated Seat Posture:**

- Sit upstanding and hurry forward on your seat.
- Raise your arms above, palms confronting one another.
- Draw in your center and lift your body somewhat off the seat, standing firm on the foothold for a couple of breaths.
- Gradually further down.

3. Seated Half Moon Posture:

- Sit upstanding with your feet level on the floor.
- Expand your right arm above, palm confronting left.
- Arrive at your left arm down towards the floor.
- Delicately twist your middle to one side, holding the posture for a couple of breaths.
- Rehash on the opposite side.

4. Seated Pigeon Posture:

- Sit with your back straight and feet on the floor.
- Get your right lower leg over your left knee.
- Incline forward marginally, keeping your back straight, to extend the stretch.
- Hold the posture for a few breaths, then switch sides.
- Props and Extras

Props can improve your seat yoga practice by offering help, security, and extra obstruction.

1.   Yoga Lash:

- Utilize a yoga lash to help with extending your arms, shoulders, and legs.
- For instance, you can fold the lash over your foot for a more profound situated ahead crease.

2.   Yoga Block:

- Utilize a yoga block for extra help during extends, for example, setting it under your foot during situated leg extends.

3.   Resistance Groups:

- Integrate opposition groups into your training to add strength preparing works out.
- For example, utilize a band around your knees for situated leg expansions.

4.   Bolster or Pad:

- Place a reinforce or pad despite your good faith for extra help during situated presents.

Seat Yoga Streams with Props

Join progressed stances and props in streaming successions for a balanced and dynamic practice.

1.   **Flow with Yoga Lash:**

- Utilize a yoga lash to help with situated ahead folds and leg extends.
- Join postures, for example, situated feline cow, side twists, and knee-to-chest extends.

2.   **Flow with Yoga Block:**

- Utilize a yoga block to improve equilibrium and soundness in stances, for example, situated seat present.
- Integrate stances like situated turn and forward overlap.

3.   **Flow with Obstruction Groups:**

- Integrate obstruction groups for added strength preparing during arm and leg works out.
- Consolidate stances, for example, situated arm circles, leg augmentations, and situated feline cow.

Redoing Seat Yoga

Find ways of redoing your seat yoga practice in view of your particular objectives, requirements, and impediments.

1.   Personalized Groupings:

- Make your own groupings by joining progressed postures and streams that line up with your objectives.

2.   Listening to Your Body:

- Continuously pay attention to your body and change acts like expected to keep away from distress or injury.

3.   Adapting Props:

- Try different things with various props and assistants to find what turns out best for your training.

4.   Setting Goals:

- Set explicit expectations for each training meeting, like further developing adaptability or developing care.

By investigating progressed seat yoga practices and figuring out how to integrate props and extras, you can develop your training and proceed with your excursion toward health. Make sure to stand by listening to your body, change acts like required, and make successions that line up with your objectives. In the following part, you'll investigate how to make a seat yoga routine for day to day practice and how to keep tabs on your development. We should proceed with your excursion to health!

CHAPTER FIVE

CREATING A DAILY CHAIR YOGA ROUTINE AND TRACKING PROGRESS

In this chapter, you will learn how to create a daily chair yoga routine that fits your needs and goals. Establishing a consistent practice is key to experiencing the benefits of chair yoga. Additionally, we'll discuss methods for tracking your progress and making adjustments to your routine as needed.

Overview:

- **Designing Your Daily Routine:** Learn how to design a chair yoga routine tailored to your goals and schedule.

- **Morning Routine:** Explore chair yoga practices for an energizing morning routine.

- **Midday Routine:** Discover chair yoga exercises to keep you focused and relaxed throughout the day.

- **Evening Routine:** Find calming chair yoga poses to unwind and prepare for a restful night's sleep.

- **Tracking Progress:** Understand how to monitor your progress and adjust your practice for continued improvement.

- **Tips for Consistency:** Gain strategies for staying committed to your chair yoga practice.

Designing Your Daily Routine

A daily chair yoga routine can be as short as 5-10 minutes or as long as 30-45 minutes, depending on your availability and goals. Consider the following steps to create a routine that suits your needs:

1. **Set Your Goals:** Determine your primary goals for practicing chair yoga, such as improving flexibility, balance, or relaxation.

2. **Choose a Time:** Decide when you want to practice chair yoga—morning, midday, or evening. Choose a time that fits into your schedule and is most conducive to your goals.

3. **Select Poses and Flows:** Based on your goals, select poses and flows that target the areas you want to focus on.

4. **Determine the Duration:** Decide how long you want your routine to be. Aim for at least 10-15 minutes per session to experience the benefits of chair yoga.

5. **Create a Sequence:** Arrange your chosen poses and flows into a sequence that is logical and aligns with your goals.

6. **Listen to Your Body:** Adjust your routine as needed based on how your body feels. Modify poses and flows if necessary.

Morning Routine

A morning chair yoga routine can help you start your day with energy and focus.

1. **Seated Breathing Exercises:**

   - Begin your routine with diaphragmatic breathing for 1-2 minutes.

2. **Seated Cat-Cow Stretch:**

   - Perform seated cat-cow stretches to warm up your spine.

   - Repeat for 5 breaths.

3. **Seated Side Bends:**

   - Reach your arm overhead and bend to each side.

   - Hold each stretch for a couple of breaths.

   - Perform 3 sets on each side.

4. **Seated Torso Twists:**

   - Twist your torso to each side, holding the stretch for a few breaths.

   - Perform 3 sets on each side.

5. **Seated Knee-to-Chest Stretch:**

   - Lift each knee to your chest and hold for a few breaths.

   - Perform 3 sets on each side.

6. **Seated Arm Circles:**

   - Extend your arms out to the sides and circle them forward and backward for 10-15 seconds each.

   - Repeat 2-3 times.

7. **Seated Forward Fold:**

   - Finish your daily schedule with a situated ahead crease.

   - Hold the stretch for several breaths before slowly rolling back up.

Midday Routine

A midday chair yoga routine can help you maintain focus and manage stress throughout the day.

1. **Seated Breathing Exercises:**

   - Begin with diaphragmatic breathing or alternate nostril breathing for 1-2 minutes.

2. **Seated Shoulder Rolls:**

   - Perform shoulder rolls to release tension in your shoulders.

   - Roll forward and backward for 10-15 seconds each.

3. **Seated Arm Stretches:**

   - Stretch your arms across your chest and behind your head.

   - • Hold each stretch for a couple of breaths.

4. **Seated Torso Twists:**

   - Twist your torso to each side, holding the stretch for a few breaths.

   - Perform 3 sets on each side.

5. **Seated Hip Stretch:**

   - Cross your right ankle over your left knee and hold the stretch for a few breaths.

   - Repeat on the other side.

   - Perform 3 sets on each side.

6. **Seated Figure Four Stretch:**

   - Perform seated figure four stretch, holding for a few breaths on each side.

7. **Seated Side Bends:**

   - Finish with seated side bends to release tension in your back and sides.

   - Hold each stretch for a couple of breaths..

Evening Routine

An evening chair yoga routine can help you unwind and prepare for a restful night's sleep.

1. **Seated Breathing Exercises:**

   - Begin with diaphragmatic breathing for 1-2 minutes.

2. **Seated Cat-Cow Stretch:**

   - Perform seated cat-cow stretches to gently move your spine.

   - Repeat for 5 breaths.

3. **Seated Forward Fold:**

   - Hinge forward from your hips and reach towards your feet.

   - Hold the stretch for several breaths.

4. **Seated Side Bends:**

   - Reach your arm overhead and bend to each side.

- Hold each stretch for a few breaths.

5. **Seated Spinal Twist:**

    - Twist your torso to each side, holding the stretch for a few breaths.

    - Perform 3 sets on each side.

6. **Seated Knee-to-Chest Stretch:**

    - Lift each knee to your chest and hold for a few breaths.

    - Perform 3 sets on each side.

7. **Seated Breathing Exercises:**

    - Finish with alternate nostril breathing for 1-2 minutes to calm your mind and body.

Tracking Progress

Monitoring your progress can help you stay motivated and adjust your practice for continued improvement.

1. **Keep a Journal:** Record your chair yoga routine, including the poses you practice and how you feel during and after your session.

2. **Set Milestones:** Set small milestones related to your goals and track your progress towards achieving them.

3. **Reflect on Changes:** Periodically reflect on any changes in your physical and mental well-being since you started practicing chair yoga.

4. **Adjust Your Routine:** Based on your reflections and progress, adjust your routine as needed to continue meeting your goals.

Tips for Consistency

Staying committed to your chair yoga practice is essential for experiencing long-term benefits.

1. **Make It a Habit:** Practice chair yoga at the same time each day to establish a routine.

2. **Start Small:** Begin with short sessions and gradually increase the duration as you become more comfortable.

3. **Be Patient:** Progress takes time, so be patient with yourself and celebrate small achievements.

4. **Stay Motivated:** Find ways to stay motivated, such as practicing with a friend or joining a chair yoga class.

5. **Listen to Your Body:** Always listen to your body and modify your practice as needed to avoid injury.

Creating a daily chair yoga routine that aligns with your goals and schedule can help you experience the full benefits of the practice. By tracking your progress and staying consistent, you can continue to improve your physical and mental well-being. In the next chapter, you'll explore chair yoga for social connections and group settings, which can enhance your practice and overall experience. Let's continue your journey to wellness!

CHAPTER SEVEN

CHAIR YOGA FOR SOCIAL CONNECTIONS AND GROUP SETTINGS

In this chapter, you will explore the benefits of practicing chair yoga in a group setting and how it can help enhance your social connections. Practicing chair yoga with others can create a supportive community and make the experience more enjoyable. Additionally, you will learn about different group settings for chair yoga, such as classes and workshops, and how to find or create your own group.

Overview:

- **Benefits of Group Chair Yoga:** Understand the advantages of practicing chair yoga in a group setting.

- **Types of Group Settings:** Explore different group settings for chair yoga, such as classes, workshops, and virtual options.

- **Finding a Chair Yoga Group:** Learn how to find a chair yoga group in your local community or online.

- **Creating Your Own Group:** Discover how to create your own chair yoga group and invite others to join.

- **Tips for Participating in Group Chair Yoga:** Gain strategies for making the most of your group chair yoga experience.

Benefits of Group Chair Yoga

Practicing chair yoga in a group setting offers several benefits that can enhance your overall experience.

1. **Social Connections:**

   - Practicing with others provides opportunities to meet new people and build friendships.

   - Social connections can enhance your sense of belonging and well-being.

2. **Motivation and Accountability:**

   - Practicing in a group setting can boost motivation and help you stay consistent with your routine.

   - Group members can hold each other accountable and provide encouragement.

3. **Shared Experience:**

   - Practicing chair yoga with others allows you to share your experiences and learn from one another.

   - Group members can offer support and advice, enhancing your practice.

4. **Guidance and Feedback:**

   - Instructors and group members can provide guidance and feedback on your practice.

- Receiving feedback can help you improve your technique and alignment.

5. **Enhanced Enjoyment:**

   - Practicing in a group setting can make chair yoga more enjoyable and fun.

   - Group members can share laughter and positive energy.

Types of Group Settings

There are various types of group settings for practicing chair yoga, each offering its own unique experience.

1. **In-Person Classes:**

   - Join a local chair yoga class to practice with others in a face-to-face setting.

   - Classes are typically led by an instructor who provides guidance and support.

2. **Workshops and Retreats:**

   - Attend chair yoga workshops or retreats for a more immersive experience.

   - Workshops may focus on specific themes or areas of practice, while retreats offer extended time for practice and relaxation.

3. **Community Centers and Senior Centers:**

   - Many community centers and senior centers offer chair yoga classes for seniors.

   - These classes provide a welcoming environment and opportunities to connect with others.

4. **Online Classes and Groups:**

   - Participate in virtual chair yoga classes or groups if you prefer practicing from home.

   - Online options offer flexibility and access to a wider range of classes and instructors.

Finding a Chair Yoga Group

Finding a chair yoga group can be a rewarding experience that enhances your practice.

1. **Local Community Centers:**

   - Check local community centers and senior centers for chair yoga classes and groups.

2. **Yoga Studios:**

   - Many yoga studios offer chair yoga classes, so check their schedules and offerings.

3. **Online Platforms:**

   - Search online platforms for virtual chair yoga classes and groups.

   - Social media and online forums can help you connect with others interested in chair yoga.

4. **Word of Mouth:**

   - Ask friends, family, or acquaintances if they know of any chair yoga groups in your area.

5. **Health and Wellness Centers:**

   - Some health and wellness centers may offer chair yoga classes, so check with local facilities.

Creating Your Own Group

If you cannot find a chair yoga group that suits your needs, consider creating your own.

1. **Invite Friends and Family:**

   - Reach out to friends, family, or acquaintances who may be interested in practicing chair yoga together.

2. **Choose a Location:**

   - Decide on a location to practice, such as your home, a local park, or a community center.

3. **Set a Schedule:**

   - Choose a regular time for your group to meet and practice chair yoga.

4. **Find an Instructor:**

   - Consider hiring a certified chair yoga instructor to lead your group and provide guidance.

5. **Share Resources:**

   - Share yoga mats, props, and other resources with group members.

Tips for Participating in Group Chair Yoga

Making the most of your group chair yoga experience can help you fully enjoy the benefits.

1. **Be Open-Minded:**

   - Embrace the shared experience and learn from others in your group.

2. **Communicate Your Needs:**

   - Let your instructor or group members know if you have any limitations or specific needs.

3. **Engage with Others:**

   - Take the time to interact with other group members and build connections.

4. **Respect Individual Differences:**

   - Understand that everyone in the group may have different levels of experience and ability.

5. **Be Supportive:**

   - Offer encouragement and support to other group members, and be open to receiving support yourself.

Practicing chair yoga in a group setting can enhance your overall experience by providing social connections, motivation, and support. Whether you find an existing group or create your own, the shared experience can make your chair yoga practice more enjoyable and rewarding. In the next chapter, you'll explore chair yoga for mindfulness and meditation, which can deepen your practice and improve your overall well-being. Let's continue your journey to wellness!

CHAPTER EIGHT

CHAIR YOGA FOR MINDFULNESS AND MEDITATION

In this chapter, you will explore how to incorporate mindfulness and meditation into your chair yoga practice. Practicing mindfulness and meditation can deepen your connection to your body and mind, reduce stress, and enhance your overall well-being. Through guided exercises and breathing techniques, you will learn how to integrate these practices into your chair yoga routine.

Overview:

- **Understanding Mindfulness and Meditation:** Learn about the principles and benefits of mindfulness and meditation.

- **Mindful Chair Yoga Practice:** Discover how to bring mindfulness into your chair yoga practice.

- **Guided Meditation Exercises:** Explore various meditation exercises that you can practice while seated in a chair.

- **Breathing Techniques for Meditation:** Learn different breathing techniques that can enhance your meditation practice.

- **Creating a Mindful Routine:** Find tips for creating a routine that incorporates mindfulness and meditation into your chair yoga practice.

Understanding Mindfulness and Meditation

Mindfulness and meditation are practices that can enhance your chair yoga experience and improve your overall well-being.

1. **Mindfulness:**

   - Care includes focusing on the current second without judgment.

   - Practicing mindfulness can help you connect more deeply with your body and breath during chair yoga.

2. **Meditation:**

   - Meditation is a practice of focusing your mind and cultivating a state of relaxation and awareness.

   - Meditation can reduce stress, anxiety, and depression while improving mental clarity and emotional stability.

3. **Benefits of Mindfulness and Meditation:**

   - Incorporating these practices into your chair yoga routine can enhance relaxation, improve focus, and promote emotional balance.

Mindful Chair Yoga Practice

Bringing mindfulness into your chair yoga practice can help you fully experience each pose and movement.

1. **Begin with Intention:**

   - Set an intention for your practice, such as focusing on your breath or cultivating gratitude.

2. **Move Slowly and Mindfully:**

   - Practice each pose with slow, deliberate movements and pay attention to your body's sensations.

3. **Focus on Your Breath:**

   - Synchronize your movements with your breath to enhance mindfulness and awareness.

4. **Notice Your Thoughts:**

   - Observe your thoughts without judgment as you practice and gently bring your focus back to your breath or movement.

5. **End with Reflection:**

   - Take a moment to reflect on your practice and how you feel physically and mentally.

Guided Meditation Exercises

Meditation exercises can be practiced while seated in a chair, making them accessible for everyone.

1. **Body Scan Meditation:**

   - Begin seated comfortably with your back straight and feet on the floor.

   - Shut your eyes and take a couple of full breaths.

   - Starting at your toes, mentally scan your body, noticing any sensations or areas of tension.

   - Slowly work your way up to the top of your head, bringing awareness to each part of your body.

   - If you encounter tension, imagine releasing it with each exhale.

2. **Loving-Kindness Meditation:**

   - Sit serenely in your seat and shut your eyes.

   - Take a few deep breaths and focus on your heart center.

   - Imagine sending loving-kindness to yourself, repeating phrases such as "May I be happy" or "May I be healthy."

- Extend this loving-kindness to others, including loved ones, acquaintances, and even those you may have conflicts with.

- Wrap up by sending cherishing thoughtfulness to all creatures.

3. **Guided Visualization:**

- Sit comfortably and close your eyes.

- Take a few deep breaths and visualize a peaceful place, such as a beach or forest.

- Imagine yourself in this serene setting, using all your senses to fully experience the environment.

- Spend a few minutes enjoying the peacefulness and return to the present when ready.

Breathing Techniques for Meditation

Different breathing techniques can enhance your meditation practice and promote relaxation.

1. **Diaphragmatic Breathing:**

- Sit comfortably with your back straight.

- Put one hand on your chest and the other on your mid-region.

- Breathe in profoundly through your nose, permitting your mid-region to grow.

- Breathe out leisurely through your mouth, feeling your mid-region contract.

- Practice for 5-10 minutes.

- 2. Substitute Nostril Relaxing:

- Sit serenely with your back straight.

- Utilize your right thumb to close your right nostril and breathe in through your left nostril.

- Close your left nostril with your right ring finger and breathe out through your right nostril.

- Breathe in through your right nostril, close it, and breathe out through your left nostril.

- Continue alternating for 5-10 minutes.

2. **Box Breathing:**

- Sit comfortably with your back straight.

- Inhale for a count of four, hold your breath for four, exhale for four, and hold your breath out for four.

- Continue this pattern for 5-10 minutes.

Creating a Mindful Routine

Incorporate mindfulness and meditation into your chair yoga practice by creating a routine that works for you.

1. **Set a Time:**

   - Choose a specific time each day to practice mindfulness and meditation.

2. **Start with Short Sessions:**

   - Begin with short meditation sessions and gradually increase the duration as you become more comfortable.

3. **Combine with Chair Yoga:**

   - Integrate mindfulness and meditation into your chair yoga practice by focusing on your breath and awareness during poses.

4. **Keep a Journal:**

   - Record your meditation experiences and any changes you notice in your mental and emotional well-being.

5. **Be Patient with Yourself:**

   - Meditation takes practice, so be patient with yourself and avoid judging your progress.

Incorporating mindfulness and meditation into your chair yoga practice can deepen your connection to your body and mind, reduce stress, and enhance your overall well-being. By practicing guided meditation exercises and breathing techniques, you can create a mindful routine that complements your chair yoga practice. In the next chapter, you'll explore chair yoga for caregivers and how it can provide support and self-care for those in caregiving roles. Let's continue your journey to wellness!

CONCLUSION

As you reach the end of this book, you have embarked on a transformative journey through chair yoga. This practice offers numerous benefits for seniors, from enhancing flexibility and balance to promoting mental and emotional well-being. By exploring various aspects of chair yoga, from beginner-level exercises to advanced practices and the integration of mindfulness and meditation, you have discovered how chair yoga can be tailored to suit your unique needs and goals.

Practicing chair yoga regularly can lead to a profound improvement in your overall quality of life. Through mindful movements and focused breathing, you can cultivate a deeper connection to your body, gain greater awareness of your physical and emotional state, and find a sense of calm amidst life's challenges.

By exploring chair yoga in different settings, whether practicing alone, with a group, or in a virtual class, you have the opportunity to build a supportive community and share the joys of this practice with others. Additionally, chair yoga can empower you to embrace a lifestyle of self-care and wellness, offering a holistic approach to maintaining health and vitality as you age.

Remember, chair yoga is a journey of self-discovery, and every practice is an opportunity to learn more about yourself. Whether you are just beginning or continuing to deepen your practice, allow yourself the grace to move at your own pace and listen to your body. Celebrate your progress and the positive changes you experience along the way.

Thank you for joining this journey through chair yoga for seniors. May your practice continue to bring you strength, balance, and serenity, enriching your life and supporting your overall well-being. As you carry forward, may you find joy and fulfillment in every chair yoga session and embrace the many rewards this practice has to offer.